Table of Contents

Introduction

Pre-diabetes is the condition that is often seen before the onset of type II diabetes. This occurs when blood sugar levels are high, but not elevated enough to warrant a diagnosis of diabetes. There are 57 million people in the Unites States with pre-diabetes.

The normal range for fasting blood sugar is 100 mg/dL or less. If the blood sugar reaches 126 mg/dL during a fasting state the individual is considered to have diabetes. Pre-diabetes is marked by a blood sugar level between 100 and 125 mg/dL. People with pre-diabetes are at higher risk of heart disease and have a 1.5-fold risk of developing heart disease compared to people with normal blood sugar. People with diabetes have a 2- to 4-fold increased risk of heart disease. We now know that people with pre-diabetes can delay or prevent the onset of type 2 diabetes through dietary and lifestyle changes. It is estimated that around 50 percent of those diagnosed with this condition, go on to develop type 2 diabetes at some point.

Physicians usually do not prescribe medication for pre-diabetes. The typical treatment is to decrease the controllable risk factors associated with diabetes such as body weight and physical activity level. Improved blood sugar levels may be achieved through a balanced diet and regular exercise. The recommendation is non-stop exercise for 30 minutes, at least five days a week. For those who have not maintained physical fitness it is important to consult with a physician before starting an exercise program.

An Overview of a Pre-Diabetes Diet

There is no specific diet for those affected by pre-diabetes. However, a diabetes diet is appropriate for individuals affected by pre-diabetes. This includes reducing intake of sweetened beverages, high-sugar foods, fatty meats, and alcoholic beverages. However, the continued intake of healthy sources of carbohydrates such as fruit, whole grains, and vegetables is encouraged.

Vegetables and fruits are essential to a healthy diet plan. Vegetables in any form; processed, cooked, or raw, are healthful. Choose plenty of low carbohydrate vegetables such as carrots, green beans, cucumber, lettuce, and broccoli. Starchy vegetables like potatoes, winter squash, and corn are higher in carbohydrate and should be eaten in appropriate portion sizes. Grains, beans, legumes, and other carbohydrate foods should be consumed in proper portion sizes.

It is important to eat protein foods to ensure a balanced diet. Protein sources include, lean meat, chicken, fish, and egg whites. Vegetarians should consult with a registered dietitian to ensure that they are receiving enough protein to promote optimal nutrition. Low-fat dairy products, such as low-fat milk and yogurt can also be part of a pre-diabetes diet program.

Weight control by initiating a healthy diet plan and increased physical activity is an important part of preventing or delaying the onset of diabetes. Foods that should be limited or avoided include pastries, cakes, sodas, and candy. Sugar-free alternatives like diet soda may be used occasionally to increase the variety of the diet.Those with pre-diabetes should follow up with their physician regularly to monitor their condition and progress.

History

In 1997, the American Diabetes Association (ADA) established the entity of impaired fasting glucose (IFG) as a prediabetes state defined as a FPG concentration of 110–125 mg/dL (6.1–6.9 mmol/L). This criterion was adopted by the World Health Organization (WHO). In 2003, the ADA lowered the criterion for IFG to 100–125 mg/dL (5.6–6.9 mmol/L). This decision was based on the observation that many fewer persons with IFG subsequently developed diabetes than those whose prediabetes was diagnosed as impaired glucose tolerance (IGT) by a 2-hour glucose value on an OGTT of 140–199 mg/dL (7.8–11.0 mmol/L). Lowering the criterion for IFG to 100–125 mg/dL (5.6–6.9 mmol/L) enabled a similar number of people with IFG and IGT to subsequently develop diabetes, although different people might fall into the different diagnostic categories of prediabetes. The WHO did not adopt this new criterion for IFG.

In 2008, an Invited Expert Panel recommended that the diabetes community consider diagnosing diabetes with an HbA1c level of 6.5% or greater (48 mmol/mol), a value just under 3 SD above the National Health and Nutrition Examination Survey population mean. They also suggested that a HbA1c level of 6.0–6.4% (42–48 mmol/mol) (>2 SD above the population mean) mandated further testing and closer follow-up. The ADA, the European Association for the Study of Diabetes, and the International Diabetes Federation then convened an International Expert Committee and agreed with the recommendation that, based on the association of diabetic retinopathy, diabetes could be diagnosed with a HbA1c level of 6.5% or greater (48 mmol/mol), if confirmed. They further argued that because of the continuum of risk in the subdiabetic glycemic range, dichotomous subdiabetic classifications (eg, prediabetes) are inappropriate and should not be created to define a specific at-risk group. Thus, they recommended that, given the lack of an identifiable threshold at which prevention efforts should be implemented, people with HbA1c levels of 6.0% or greater (42 mmol/mol), which is obviously near the diagnostic threshold, should be monitored more closely and should be considered candidates for an intervention to prevent diabetes.

The ADA formally accepted the recommendation for the diagnosis of diabetes but went further by adopting an HbA1c criterion for prediabetes of 5.7%–6.4% (39–48 mmol/mol). The lower bounds of the HbA1c criterion for prediabetes was apparently based on the cross-sectional values of the 2005–2006 National Health and Nutrition Examination Survey population that were fed into models that estimated the risk for developing diabetes and CVD, rather than on prospective studies. The WHO accepted the ADA recommendation on the HbA1c criterion for diagnosing diabetes but believed that that there was insufficient evidence to make any recommendations for values less than 6.5% (48 mmol/mol).

As expected, using the ADA definition for prediabetes, the number of Americans potentially diagnosed with the condition is enormous, nearly 40% of the adult population. Gregg et al have pointed out that the less strict the criteria used to identify prediabetes, the more people will be eligible for an intervention, and therefore, more individuals may be helped but at the cost of a large number for whom the intervention would not be necessary because they were not destined to develop diabetes. Conversely, the more strict the criteria for prediabetes, the fewer the individuals who will be eligible for an intervention, but there would be greater economic efficiency in that more cases of diabetes would be delayed per individual receiving the intervention.

Given the trade-offs identified by Gregg et al, the observation that achieving diabetes prevention in clinical trials was expensive, and that sustainable weight loss has been very difficult to achieve in community settings, all suggest that considerable resources would be necessary to prevent/delay the development of diabetes in a population. Moreover, and at the least before initiating nationwide programs, we should critically examine the evidence that prediabetes has clinical merit. Specifically, the question is whether an FPG of 100–109 mg/dL (5.6–6.0 mmol/L) or a HbA1c of 5.7–5.9 (39–41 mmol/mol) or even an FPG of 110–125 mg/dL (6.1–6.9 mmol/L) or a HbA1c of 6.0–6.4 (42–48 mmol/mol) represent sufficient risk of a clinical adverse outcome, ie, a CVD event or a microvascular complication, after prediabetes developed into diabetes, that would merit an intervention. (Since the OGTT is rarely used in nonpregnant individuals, we only evaluate the benefit of identifying those with prediabetes by the FPG or HbA1c criteria.)

The papers on which this Position Statement is based were identified in a comprehensive review of publications from 2003 through 2015. The ADA recommended the lower glucose bounds of prediabetes in 2003 and the lower HbA1c bounds of prediabetes in 2011. Only incident studies that separately tracked the association with CVD and the development of diabetes within the lower and upper bounds of the ADA definitions of prediabetes in the same population from 2003 were reviewed. This limited the number of studies analyzed in this manuscript because the vast majority related to this subject simply tracked subjects with IGT or individuals who fulfilled the entire definitions of the ADA or the WHO. Since 1995, the first author has published 20 papers on screening for and diagnosing diabetes and has kept an extensive file in this area. Articles in this file from 2003 through 2015 and their bibliographies were reviewed, and 31 papers that fulfilled the criteria mentioned above were identified and thus were included in this Position Statement.

Prediabetes

Prediabetes is when your blood sugar level is higher than it should be but not high enough for your doctor to diagnose diabetes. They might call it impaired fasting glucose or impaired glucose tolerance.

People with type 2 diabetes almost always had prediabetes first. But it doesn't usually cause symptoms. About 84 million people over age 20 in the U.S. have prediabetes, but 90% don't know that they have it.

Prediabetes treatment can prevent more serious health problems, including type 2 diabetes and problems with your heart, blood vessels, eyes, and kidneys.

A person with borderline diabetes, or prediabetes, has blood sugar levels that are higher than normal but not yet high enough for a diagnosis of type 2 diabetes.

Borderline diabetes is a condition that may lead to type 2 diabetes. According to the American Diabetes Association, an estimated 10 to 23 percent of people with borderline diabetes will go on to develop type 2 diabetes within 5 years.

Doctors may also refer to borderline diabetes as:

- insulin resistance
- impaired glucose tolerance
- impaired fasting glucose

This book looks at how to recognize risk factors for prediabetes, how to manage the condition, and how to prevent type 2 diabetes from developing.

Symptoms

Prediabetes does not produce clear symptoms, so regular checks are important for people who are at risk.

Prediabetes does not have clear symptoms. Some people may not be aware that they have it until:

- a doctor tests blood glucose and blood pressure levels
- prediabetes has progressed to type 2 diabetes
- a complication occurs, such as a heart attack

If a person's blood sugar level remains high, they may begin to develop some symptoms of type 2 diabetes. Symptoms include frequent urination and increased thirst.

Most people will not know they have prediabetes until they receive testing.

Causes and risk factors

According to the National Institute of Diabetes and Digestive and Kidney Diseases (NIDDK), a range of other conditions can increase the risk of prediabetes, including:

- obesity, especially abdominal obesity
- high blood pressure
- high blood fat levels, or triglycerides
- low levels of "good" high-density lipoprotein (HDL) cholesterol

Other risk factors include:

- not getting enough exercise
- having a family history of type 2 diabetes.

According to the American Heart Association, the following lifestyle factors may also be a risk for prediabetes in some people:

- raised stress levels

- smoking

- drinking too much alcohol

Regularly consuming high-sugar drinks may also increase the risk.

Sugary drinks can contribute to the development of diabetes.

One 2017 review found that people who regularly drink sugary beverages face an increased risk of metabolic diseases, such as high blood pressure and high levels of blood glucose and fats.

These metabolic conditions can lead to prediabetes and diabetes.

People who lead an inactive lifestyle are at higher risk of taking in too many calories without burning them through exercise.

Other people who may be at risk of developing prediabetes include those with polycystic ovary syndrome (PCOS) and those who have experienced instances of high blood sugar levels in the past.

Anyone with any of these risk factors may benefit from a prediabetes screening to identify whether they have the condition.

A doctor typically diagnoses prediabetes with a blood test, particularly a glucose tolerance test. A glucose tolerance test measures how quickly the body can process the sugar in the blood in a 2-hour period.

Other tests include measuring blood sugar levels after a person has not eaten for a specific period. This is called a fasting blood test.

The doctor may also use an A1C test. This involves measuring the average blood sugar levels over 2–3 months. People do not need to fast or take any special liquids or medications for this test, and it gives reliable results.

According to the American Diabetes Association, a doctor will diagnose prediabetes when test results show the following measurements:

- fasting blood sugar levels of 100–125 milligrams per deciliter (mg/dl)
- glucose tolerance levels of 140–199 mg/dl
- an A1C test result of 5.7–6.4 percent

A doctor will often re-test these levels to confirm that the readings are not due to one-off spikes in blood sugar.

Blood glucose monitors for home use are available for purchase online.

Who should seek screening?

The NIDDK recommend that people with the following risk factors should undergo a prediabetes screening:

- an age of 45 years or over
- obesity or overweight, or a body mass index (BMI) over 25
- a waist circumference larger than 40 inches in males or over 35 inches in females
- a close relative with diabetes
- a condition that increases insulin resistance, including PCOS, acanthosis nigricans, and nonalcoholic steatohepatitis
- an ethnic background that places an individual at high risk of diabetes, including people who are African-American, Asian-American, Latino, Native American, or a Pacific Islander

- a history of gestational diabetes, or diabetes as a result of pregnancy
- having given birth to an infant weighing over 9 pounds
- having a disease that harden the arteries
- recent treatment with glucocorticoids or atypical antipsychotic medications

If a doctor identifies any of these risk factors, they may recommend that the person has a screening for blood glucose levels.

Medical professionals advise repeating screening tests every 1 to 3 years if a person has these risk factors.

The NIDDK has an official resource to check diabetes risk.

However, anyone who is concerned that they may have borderline diabetes should visit the doctor for testing and a proper diagnosis.

How diet relates to prediabetes

There are many factors that increase your risk for prediabetes. Genetics can play a role, especially if diabetes runs in your family. However, other factors play a larger role in the development of disease. Inactivity and having overweight are other potential risk factors.

In prediabetes, sugar from food begins to build up in your bloodstream because insulin can't easily move it into your cells.

People think of carbohydrate as the culprit that causes prediabetes, but the amount and type of carbohydrates consumed in a meal is what influences blood sugar. A diet filled with refined and processed carbohydrates that digest quickly can cause higher spikes in blood sugar.

For most people with prediabetes, the body has a difficult time lowering blood sugar levels after meals. Avoiding blood sugar spikes by watching your carbohydrate intake can help.

When you eat more calories than your body needs, they get stored as fat. This can cause you to gain weight. Body fat, especially around the belly, is linked to insulin resistance. This explains why many people with prediabetes also have overweight.

Healthy eating

You can't control all risk factors for prediabetes, but some can be mitigated. Lifestyle changes can help you maintain balanced blood sugar levels and stay within a healthy weight range.

The glycemic index (GI) is a tool you can use to determine how a particular food could affect your blood sugar.

Foods that are high on the GI will raise your blood sugar faster. Foods ranked lower on the scale have less effect on your blood sugar spike. Foods with high fiber are low on the GI. Foods that are processed, refined, and void of fiber and nutrients register high on the GI.

Refined carbohydrates rank high on the GI. These are grain products that digest quickly in your stomach. Examples are white bread, russet potatoes, and white rice, along with soda and juice. Limit these foods whenever possible if you have prediabetes.

Foods that rank medium on the GI are fine to eat. Examples include whole-wheat bread and brown rice. Still, they aren't as good as foods that rank low on the GI.

Foods that are low on the GI are best for your blood sugar. Incorporate the following items in your diet:

- steel-cut oats (not instant oatmeal)

- stone-ground whole wheat bread

- nonstarchy vegetables, such as carrots and field greens

- beans

- sweet potatoes

- corn

- pasta (preferably whole wheat)

Food and nutrition labels don't reveal the GI of a given item. Instead make note of the fiber content listed on the label to help determine a food's GI ranking.

Remember to limit saturated fat intake to reduce the risk of developing high cholesterol and heart disease, along with prediabetes.

Eating mixed meals is a great way to lower a food's given GI. For example, if you plan to eat white rice, add vegetables and chicken to slow down the digestion of the grain and minimize spikes.

Portion control

Good portion control can keep your diet on the low GI. This means you limit the amount of food you eat. Often, portions in the United States are much larger than intended serving sizes. A bagel serving size is usually about one-half, yet many people eat the whole bagel.

Food labels can help you determine how much you're eating. The label will list calories, fat, carbohydrates, and other nutrition information for a particular serving.

If you eat more than the serving listed, it's important to understand how that'll affect the nutritional value. A food may have 20 grams of carbohydrate and 150

calories per serving. But if you have two servings, you've consumed 40 grams of carbohydrate and 300 calories.

Eliminating carbohydrates altogether isn't necessary. Recent research has shown that a lower carb diet (less than 40 percent carbs) is associated with the same mortality risk increase as a high carbohydrate diet (greater than 70 percent carbs).

The study noted minimal risk observed when consuming 50 to 55 percent carbohydrates in a day. On a 1600-calorie diet, this would equal 200 grams of carbohydrates daily. Spreading intake out evenly throughout the day is best.

This is in line with the National Institutes of Health and the Mayo Clinic's recommendation of 45 to 65 percent of calories coming from carbohydrates daily. Individual carbohydrate needs will vary based on a person's stature and activity level.

Speaking to a dietitian about specific needs is recommended.

One of the best methods to manage portions is to practice mindful eating. Eat when you're hungry. Stop when you're full. Sit, and eat slowly. Focus on the food and flavors.

Eating more fiber-rich foods

Fiber offers several benefits. It helps you feel fuller, longer. Fiber adds bulk to your diet, making bowel movements easier to pass.

Eating fiber-rich foods can make you less likely to overeat. They also help you avoid the "crash" that can come from eating a high sugar food. These types of foods will often give you a big boost of energy, but make you feel tired shortly after.

Examples of high-fiber foods include:

- beans and legumes
- fruits and vegetables that have an edible skin
- whole grain breads

- whole grains, such as quinoa or barley
- whole grain cereals
- whole wheat pasta
- Cut out sugary drinks

A single, 12-ounce can of soda can contain 45 grams of carbohydrates. That number is the recommended carbohydrate serving for a meal for women with diabetes.

Sugary sodas only offer empty calories that translate to quick-digesting carbohydrates. Water is a better choice to quench your thirst.

Drink alcohol in moderation

Moderation is a healthy rule to live by in most instances. Drinking alcohol is no exception. Many alcoholic beverages are dehydrating. Some cocktails may contain high sugar levels that can spike your blood sugar.

According to the Dietary Guidelines for Americans, women should only have one drink per day, while men should limit themselves to no more than two drinks per day.

Drink servings relate back to portion control. The following are the measurements for an average single drink:

- 1 bottle of beer (12 fluid ounces)

- 1 glass of wine (5 fluid ounces)

- 1 shot of distilled spirits, such as gin, vodka, or whiskey (1.5 fluid ounces)

Keep your drink as simple as possible. Avoid adding sugary juices or liqueurs. Keep a glass of water nearby that you can sip on to prevent dehydration.

Eat lean meats

Meat doesn't contain carbohydrates, but it can be a significant source of saturated fat in your diet. Eating a lot of fatty meat can lead to high cholesterol levels.

If you have prediabetes, a diet low in saturated fat and trans fat can help reduce your risk of heart disease. It's recommended that you avoid cuts of meat with visible fat or skin.

Choose protein sources such as the following:

- chicken without skin

- egg substitute or egg whites

- beans and legumes

- soybean products, such as tofu and tempeh

- fish, such as cod, flounder, haddock, halibut, tuna, or trout
- lean beef cuts, such as flank steak, ground round, tenderloin, and roast with fat trimmed
- shellfish, such as crab, lobster, shrimp, or scallops
- turkey without skin
- low fat Greek yogurt

Very lean cuts of meat have about 0 to 1 gram of fat and 35 calories per ounce. High-fat meat choices, such as spareribs, can have more than 7 grams of fat and 100 calories per ounce.

Drinking plenty of water

Water is an important part of any healthy diet. Drink enough water each day to keep you from becoming dehydrated. If you have prediabetes, water is a healthier alternative than sugary sodas, juices, and energy drinks.

The amount of water you should drink every day depends on your body size, activity level, and the climate you live in.

You can determine if you're drinking enough water by monitoring the volume of urine when you go. Also make note of the color. Your urine should be pale yellow.

Exercise and diet go together

Exercise is a part of any healthy lifestyle. It's especially important for those with prediabetes.

A lack of physical activity has been linked to increased insulin resistance, according to the National Institute of Diabetes and Digestive and Kidney Diseases (NIDDK). Exercise causes muscles to use glucose for energy, and makes the cells work more effectively with insulin.

The NIDDK recommends exercising 5 days a week for at least 30 minutes. Exercise doesn't have to be strenuous or overly complicated. Walking, dancing, riding a bicycle, taking an exercise class, or finding another activity you enjoy are all examples of physical activity.

Breaking the prediabetes chain

The Centers for Disease Control and Prevention (CDC) estimate that 84 million U.S. adults have prediabetes. Perhaps even more concerning is that 90 percent don't know they have the condition.

Early medical intervention is important in order to catch the condition before it turns into type 2 diabetes. If you've been diagnosed with prediabetes, you and your doctor can develop a diet plan that will help.

Best And Worst Foods For Diabetes

Your food choices matter a lot when you've got diabetes. Some are better than others.

Nothing is completely off-limits. Even items that you might think of as "the worst" could be occasional treats -- in tiny amounts. But they won't help you nutrition-wise, and it's easiest to manage your diabetes if you mainly stick to the "best" options.

Starches

Your body needs carbs. But you want to choose wisely. Use this list as a guide.

Best Choices

Whole grains, such as brown rice, oatmeal, quinoa, millet, or amaranth

Baked sweet potato

Items made with whole grains and no (or very little) added sugar

Worst Choices

Processed grains, such as white rice or white flour

Cereals with little whole grains and lots of sugar

White bread

French fries

Fried white-flour tortillas

Vegetables

Load up! You'll get fiber and very little fat or salt (unless you add them). Remember, potatoes and corn count as carbs.

Best Choices

Fresh veggies, eaten raw or lightly steamed, roasted, or grilled

Plain frozen vegetables, lightly steamed

Greens such as kale, spinach, and arugula. Iceberg lettuce is not as great because it's low in nutrients.

Low sodium or unsalted canned vegetables

Go for a variety of colors: dark greens, red or orange (think of carrots or red peppers), whites (onions) and even purple (eggplants). The 2015 U.S. guidelines recommend 2.5 cups of veggies per day.

Worst Choices

Canned vegetables with lots of added sodium

Veggies cooked with lots of added butter, cheese, or sauce

Pickles, if you need to limit sodium. Otherwise, pickles are OK.

Sauerkraut, for the same reason as pickles. Limit them if you have high blood pressure.

Fruits

They give you carbohydrates, vitamins, minerals, and fiber. Most are naturally low in fat and sodium. But they tend to have more carbs than vegetables do.

Best Choices

Fresh fruit

Plain frozen fruit or fruit canned without added sugar

Sugar-free or low-sugar jam or preserves

No-sugar-added applesauce

Worst Choices

Canned fruit with heavy sugar syrup

Chewy fruit rolls

Regular jam, jelly, and preserves (unless you have a very small portion)

Sweetened applesauce

Fruit punch, fruit drinks, fruit juice drinks

Top Picks

Protein

You have lots of choices, including beef, chicken, fish, pork, turkey, seafood, beans, cheese, eggs, nuts, and tofu.

Best Choices

The American Diabetes Association lists these as the top options:

Plant-based proteins such as beans, nuts, seeds, or tofu

Fish and seafood

Chicken and other poultry (Choose the breast meat if possible.)

Eggs and low-fat dairy

If you eat meat, keep it low in fat. Trim the skin off of poultry.

Try to include some plant-based protein from beans, nuts, or tofu, even if you're not a vegetarian or vegan. You'll get nutrients and fiber that aren't in animal products.

Worst Choices

Fried meats

Higher-fat cuts of meat, such as ribs

Pork bacon

Regular cheeses

Poultry with skin

Deep-fried fish

Deep-fried tofu

Beans prepared with lard

Dairy

Keep it low in fat. If you want to splurge, keep your portion small.

Best Choices

1% or skim milk

Low-fat yogurt

Low-fat cottage cheese

Low-fat or nonfat sour cream

Worst Choices

Whole milk

Regular yogurt

Regular cottage cheese

Regular sour cream

Regular ice cream

Regular half-and-half

Fats, Oils, and Sweets

They're tough to resist. But it's easy to get too much and gain weight, which makes it harder to manage your diabetes.

Best Choices

Natural sources of vegetable fats, such as nuts, seeds, or avocados (high in calories, so keep portions small)

Foods that give you omega-3 fatty acids, such as salmon, tuna, or mackerel

Plant-based oils, such as canola, grapeseed, or olive oils

Worst Choices

Anything with trans fat in it. It's bad for your heart. Check the ingredient list for anything that's "partially hydrogenated," even if the label says it has 0 grams of trans fat.

Big portions of saturated fats, which mainly come from animal products but also are in coconut oil and palm oil. Ask your doctor what your limit should be, especially if you have heart disease as well as diabetes.

Drinks

When you down a favorite drink, you may get more calories, sugar, salt, or fat than you bargained for. Read the labels so you know what's in a serving.

Best Choices

Unflavored water or flavored sparkling water

Unsweetened tea with or without a slice of lemon

Light beer, small amounts of wine, or non-fruity mixed drinks

Coffee, black or with added low-fat milk and sugar substitute

Worst Choices

Regular sodas

Regular beer, fruity mixed drinks, dessert wines

Sweetened tea

Coffee with sugar and cream

Flavored coffees and chocolate drinks

Energy drinks

Recipes

Low-fat roasties

Ingredients

800g roasting potatoes, quartered

1 garlic clove, sliced

200ml vegetable stock (from a cube is fine)

2 tbsp olive oil

Method

Heat oven to 200C/fan 180C/gas 6. Put the potatoes and garlic in a roasting tin. Pour over the stock, then brush the tops of the potatoes with half the olive oil. Season, then cook for 50 mins. Brush with the remaining oil and cook 10-15 mins more until the stock is absorbed and the potatoes have browned and cooked through.

Caramelised carrots & onions

Ingredients

500g carrot, peeled and cut into long chunks

50g butter

1 tbsp olive oil

8 red onions, peeled and quartered with root intact

3 sprigs thyme

1 tbsp soft brown sugar

3 tbsp red wine

1 tbsp good-quality balsamic vinegar

Method

Blanch carrots in a pan of boiling salted water for 3 mins, drain well, then pat dry. In a large pan, melt the butter and oil, then fry the carrots, onions and thyme over a low heat for 30 mins until golden.

Stir in the sugar and red wine and bubble for a few mins to boil off the alcohol. Add the vinegar, then continue to cook until syrupy, about 5 mins. Remove the sprigs of thyme and serve. Make up to 2 days ahead, stored in a covered container. Tip back into a pan and reheat or use a microwave.

Leftover turkey casserole

Ingredients

2 onions, finely chopped

1 eating apple, cored and chopped

2 tbsp olive oil

1 tsp dried sage, or 5 sage leaves, chopped

2 tbsp plain flour

300ml vegetable or chicken stock

2 tbsp wholegrain mustard

2 tbsp runny honey

400g-500g leftover turkey, shredded

about 350g leftover roasted vegetables like roast potatoes, parsnips, celeriacs and carrots, chunkily diced

Method

Fry the onion and apple in the oil until softened in a casserole or deep pan. Stir in the sage for 1 min, then stir in the flour. Gradually stir in the stock followed by the mustard and honey.

Bring up to a simmer and stir in the turkey and roast veg. Cover and gently simmer for 15 mins until turkey is piping hot. Season and eat with mash or jacket potatoes.

Turkey & parsnip curry

Ingredients

2 tbsp vegetable oil

2 onions, halved through the root and thinly sliced

500g parsnip, peeled and cut into chunks

5 tbsp Madras curry paste

400g can chopped tomatoes

500g/1lb 2oz boneless cooked turkey, cut into chunks

150g pot low-fat natural yogurt

cooked basmati rice, to serve

Method

Heat the oil in a saucepan, add the onions and fry gently for 10 minutes until they are softened and lightly coloured. Add the parsnips and stir well.

To make the curry, stir in the curry paste, then add the tomatoes with a little salt, and stir well. Add 1½ canfuls of water and bring to the boil. Reduce the heat, cover and simmer for 15-20 minutes, until the parsnips are just tender.

To finish, stir in the turkey chunks, cover the pan again and simmer for a further 5 minutes until the turkey is heated through. Remove from the heat. (The curry can now be cooled and frozen for up to 2 months.) Lightly swirl in the yogurt and serve with basmati rice.

Pan-fried venison with blackberry sauce

Ingredients

1 tbsp olive oil

2 thick venison

steaks, or 4 medallions

1 tbsp balsamic vinegar

150ml beef stock (made with 2 tsp Knorr Touch of Taste beef concentrate)

2 tbsp redcurrant jelly

1 garlic clove, crushed

85g fresh or frozen blackberry

Method

Heat the oil in a frying pan, cook the venison for 5 mins, then turn over and cook for 3-5 mins more, depending on how rare you like it and the thickness of the meat (cook for 5-6 mins on each side for well done). Lift the meat from the pan and set aside to rest.

Add the balsamic vinegar to the pan, then pour in the stock, redcurrant jelly and garlic. Stir over quite a high heat to blend everything together, then add the blackberries and carry on cooking until they soften. Serve with the venison, celeriac mash (see below) and broccoli.

Chargrilled vegetable salad

Ingredients

2 red peppers

3 tbsp olive oil

1 tbsp red wine vinegar

1 small garlic clove, crushed

1 red chilli, deseeded, finely chopped

1 aubergine, cut into 1cm rounds

2 red onions, sliced about 1½ cm thick but kept as whole slices

6 plump sundried tomatoes in oil, drained and torn into strips

handful black olives

large handful basil, roughly torn

Method

First, blacken the peppers all over – do this directly over a flame, over hot coals or under a hot grill. When completely blackened, put them in a bowl, cover with a plate and leave to cool.

While the peppers are cooling, mix the oil, vinegar, garlic and chilli in a large bowl. On a hot barbecue or griddle pan, chargrill the aubergine, courgette and onions in batches until they have defined grill marks on both sides and are starting to soften. The time will depend on the intensity of your grill, so use your judgement – courgettes and red onions are fine still slightly crunchy but you want the aubergine cooked all the way through. As the vegetables are ready, put them straight into the dressing to marinate, breaking the onions up into rings.

When the peppers are cool enough to handle, peel, remove the stalk and scrape out the seeds. Cut into strips and toss through the veg with any juice from the bowl. Mix in the tomatoes, olives, basil and seasoning. Drizzle with more oil, if you like, and serve either on its own or with mozzarella or crumbled feta.

Make-ahead mushroom soufflés

Ingredients

140g small button mushroom, sliced

50g butter, plus extra for greasing

25g plain flour

325ml milk

85g gruyère, finely grated, plus a little extra

3 large eggs, separated

6 tsp crème fraîche

snipped chive, to serve

Method

Fry the mushrooms in the butter for about 3 mins, then remove from the heat and reserve a good spoonful. Add the flour to the rest, then blend in the milk and return to the heat, stirring all the time to make a thick sauce. Stir in the cheese, season to taste, then leave to cool.

Heat oven to 200C/fan 180C/gas 6. Butter 8 x 150ml soufflé dishes and line the bases with baking paper. Stir the egg yolks into the soufflé mixture, then whisk the egg whites until stiff before folding in carefully. Spoon into the soufflé dishes and bake in a roasting tin, half-filled with cold water, for 15 mins until risen and golden. Leave to cool (they will sink, but they are meant to). You can make the soufflés up to this stage up to 2 days ahead. Cover and chill.

When ready to serve, turn the soufflés out of their dishes, peel off the lining paper, then put them on a baking sheet lined with small squares of baking paper. Top each soufflé with 1 tsp crème fraîche and a little cheese, then scatter with the reserved mushrooms. Bake at 190C/fan 170C/gas 5 for 10-15 mins until slightly risen and warmed through. Sprinkle with chives and serve.

Braised sea bass with spinach

Ingredients

2 red peppers, halved, deseeded

2 tbsp extra-virgin olive oil, plus extra for drizzling

2 shallots, chopped

1 garlic clove, finely chopped

250g cherry or baby plum tomato, halved

small handful capers

12 large black olives, stoned and roughly chopped

20 basil leaves

50ml white wine

100ml/3½ fl oz tomato juice

2 whole sea bass, about 600-700g/1lb 5oz-1lb-9oz each, gutted, scaled and cleaned (get your fishmonger to do this)

large knob butter

250g bag spinach

Method

Heat the grill to high. Put the peppers, skin side up, on a baking tray, then pop them under the hot grill for about 10 mins until the skins blister and blacken. Drop them into a bowl, cover with some cling film and leave until cool enough to handle. Peel away and discard the skins, then roughly chop the peppers.

Heat the oil over a low-ish heat in a sturdy roasting tin or in a shallow pan that has a lid and is large enough to fit both fish. Throw in the shallots and garlic and sweat briefly until soft. Stir in the tomatoes, peppers, capers, olives and half the basil leaves, then sweat for a few mins until the tomatoes soften. Pour in the wine and tomato juice. Stir and gently simmer for 10-15 mins, adding a splash of water if the sauce becomes a bit dry.

While the sauce is simmering, slash each side of the fish a few times. When the sauce is ready lay the fish on top, season if you want to and cover with a lid (cover with foil if you are using a roasting tray). Leave to cook on a low heat for 12-15 mins until the flesh feels firm when pressed.

While the fish is cooking, melt the butter in a large pan, then fry the spinach until wilted, season if you like and divide the spinach between two serving dishes. Lift the fish carefully from the pan and place on top of the spinach, neatly drizzle some of the sauce round the fish, scatter the remaining basil on top and drizzle everything with extra-virgin olive oil. Serve with some ribbon shaped pasta, like tagliatelle or pappardelle, with the remaining sauce in a bowl or side dish.

Grilled goat's cheese with cranberry dressing

Ingredients

2 red-skinned apples

3 tbsp lemon juice

3 x 100g Capricorn goat's cheese, halved horizontally

2 tbsp cranberry jelly

2 tbsp olive oil

1 tsp clear honey

25g pecan

2 chicory

heads, separated into leaves

handful radish sprouts (available from larger supermarkets) or watercress

Method

Quarter, core, then thinly slice the apple into a bowl with the lemon juice and 1 tbsp water. Toss well, as this stops the apples going brown.

Heat grill to high, then line your grill rack with foil. Put the cheeses rind-side down on the foil, then set aside for a moment.

Drain 2 tbsp of the juice from the apple bowl into another small bowl and discard the rest. Add the cranberry sauce, oil and honey with some seasoning, and whisk to form a dressing. Grill the cheeses for 4 mins, then scatter the nuts on and around the cheeses and return to the grill to cook for a few mins more – but take care that the nuts don't burn.

Arrange the apple, chicory and radish sprouts or watercress on 6 plates, then carefully top with the hot melted cheese. Scatter over the nuts, spoon over the dressing and serve straight away.

Spiced carrot & lentil soup

Ingredients

2 tsp cumin seeds

pinch chilli flakes

2 tbsp olive oil

600g carrots, washed and coarsely grated (no need to peel)

140g split red lentils

1l hot vegetable stock (from a cube is fine)

125ml milk

(to make it dairy-free, see 'try' below)

plain yogurt

and naan bread, to serve

Method

Heat a large saucepan and dry-fry 2 tsp cumin seeds and a pinch of chilli flakes for 1 min, or until they start to jump around the pan and release their aromas.

Scoop out about half with a spoon and set aside. Add 2 tbsp olive oil, 600g coarsely grated carrots, 140g split red lentils, 1l hot vegetable stock and 125ml milk to the pan and bring to the boil.

Simmer for 15 mins until the lentils have swollen and softened.

Whizz the soup with a stick blender or in a food processor until smooth (or leave it chunky if you prefer).

Season to taste and finish with a dollop of plain yogurt and a sprinkling of the reserved toasted spices. Serve with warmed naan breads.

Juicy Lucy pudding

Ingredients

350g packet frozen fruits of the forest, defrosted

3 tbsp light muscovado sugar

4 tbsp no-added-sugar wild blueberry

jam (we used St Dalfour, from larger supermarket branches)

6 medium-sized ripe pears, peeled, quartered and cored

50g fresh white breadcrumb

25g butter, melted

Method

Preheat the oven to 190C/gas 5/ fan 170C. Mix the fruits of the forest in a large bowl with the sugar and jam, then add the pears and toss to mix. Tip into a deep baking dish measuring about 18x28cm, cover with foil and roast in the oven for 20 minutes. Pierce a pear or two to see if they are really tender; if not, return dish to the oven for another 5 minutes or until they feel soft.

Mix breadcrumbs with the butter and scatter over the fruit. Bake uncovered in the oven for 10-15 minutes or until golden and crispy. Serve hot.

Prawn & fennel bisque

Ingredients

450g raw tiger prawn in their shells

4 tbsp olive oil

1 large onion, chopped

1 large fennel bulb, chopped, fronds reserved

2 carrots, chopped

150ml dry white wine

1 tbsp brandy

400g can chopped tomato

1l fish stock

2 generous pinches paprika

To serve

150ml pot double cream

8 tiger prawns, shelled, but tail tips left on (optional)

fennel fronds (optional)

Method

Shell the prawns, then fry the shells in the oil in a large pan for about 5 mins. Add the onion, fennel and carrots and cook for about 10 mins until the veg start to soften. Pour in the wine and brandy, bubble hard for about 1 min to drive off the alcohol, then add the tomatoes, stock and paprika. Cover and simmer for 30 mins. Meanwhile, chop the prawns.

Blitz the soup as finely as you can with a stick blender or food processor, then press through a sieve into a bowl. Spend a bit of time really working the mixture through the sieve as this will give the soup its velvety texture.

Tip back into a clean pan, add the prawns and cook for 10 mins, then blitz again until smooth. You can make and chill this a day ahead or freeze it for 1 month. Thaw ovenight in the fridge. To serve, gently reheat in a pan with the cream. If garnishing, cook the 8 prawns in a little butter. Spoon into small bowls and top with the prawns and snipped fennel fronds.

Mushroom & thyme risotto

Ingredients

1 tbsp olive oil

350g chestnut mushrooms, sliced

100g quinoa

1l hot vegetable stock

175g risotto rice

handful of thyme leaves

handful of grated parmesan

or vegetarian alternative

50g bag rocket, to serve

Method

Heat the oil in a medium pan, sauté the mushrooms for 2-3 mins, then stir in the quinoa. Keeping the vegetable stock warm in a separate pan on a low heat, add a ladle of the stock and stir until absorbed. Stir in the rice and repeat again with the stock, until all the stock has been used up and the rice and quinoa are tender and cooked.

Stir in the thyme leaves, then divide between four plates or bowls. Serve topped with grated parmesan and rocket leaves.

Conclusion

In conclusion, a prediabetes state could potentially have a similar impact as diabetes on coronary and peripheral atherosclerosis. Larger studies are needed in the prediabetes population to establish a direct link between prediabetes and CAD.